HOW TO ACHIEVE A LIFE EXPERIENCE WITHOUT LIMITATIONS

VICTOR MANUEL ARREOLA C.

BARKER JULES

BARKER & JULES®

How to achieve a life experience without limitations

Edition: Miguel Moreno | BARKER & JULES™
Book cover design by Paulina López | BARKER & JULES™
Book interior layout by Paulina López | BARKER & JULES™

All rights reserved. © 2023, by Victor Manuel Arreola C.

First Edition. Published by BARKER & JULES®

I.S.B.N. Paperback | 979-8-88929-108-4
I.S.B.N. Hardback | 979-8-88929-109-1
I.S.B.N. eBook | 979-8-88929-107-7

Library of Congress Copyrights Control Number: 1-12038867051

Printed in the United States.

BARKER & JULES® and their affiliates are an imprint of BARKER & JULES, LLC.

BARKER & JULES, LLC
500 Broadway 606, Santa Monica, CA 90401
barkerandjules.com

HOW TO ACHIEVE A LIFE EXPERIENCE WITHOUT LIMITATIONS

VICTOR MANUEL ARREOLA C.

BARKER JULES

Acknowledgments

First of all, I want to thank my creator, the almighty, the creator of life: and to my family, my wife, son and daughter, I also want to dedicate this piece of work to a very special person who always showed himself to the world with open arms; Jose de Jesus, "Chuyito", as many of us called him, a person who is no longer with us, but his natural essence will remain present.

His love for life, his simplicity and nobility towards others left behind a legacy in the lives of those who knew him. Undoubtedly, he taught us how to live life without limitations, without thinking what people will say, what they will think, to become a free person on the inside, free of everything that limits us to achieve great goals. One day before leaving this world, Chuyito achieved one of his greatest goals, to win a medal in the sport of weightlifting. He fought for everything he set out to achieve.

He always sought to put a smile on the faces of others, doing the impossible to be accepted as he was, with his defects and limitations, but also with his greatness as a human being that characterized him and made him different from others.
The day of his funeral, his family and friends shared

how he left a lasting memory in their lives. This made me reflect that if we all were like Chuyito was, the world would be different, for him there was no evil, resentment, or hatred, he just wanted to be happy and live his life to its fullest, surrounded by his family and friends.

Making other people happy filled him with inner satisfaction, his father, mother, sisters, family, and friends were everything to him, he definitely knew how to live life to the fullest, with its ups and downs. We cannot deny that he also experienced feelings and emotions like every human being, he learned to smile, cry, experience anger and resentment, but he did not perpetuate those feelings because the most important thing for him was undoubtedly love, forgiveness and serving others. These were just some of his qualities that made him different from everyone else.

He, at thirty-three years old, left behind a legacy and a lesson for humanity and that is why I want to leave a little of his story in these letters. Chuyito did not die, he simply transformed into what each one of us really are and someday we will share that same transformation. His mission was to serve others and to be happy.

RIP José de Jesús Arreola (Chuyito)
7/24/1989 - 8/07/2022

Arreola Professional Services INC.
DBA: VMA Publications
Rialto, Ca. 92376
victormanuelarreola.com

Foreword

For centuries, mankind has devoted itself to the search for some method of attaining eternal happiness. Day after day we run from one place to another without knowing what we are really looking for, we think and take for granted that happiness is everything, and we are willing to give our lives to achieve it. It is necessary to understand that there is a difference between "**happiness**" and "**emotional psychological well-being**".

Developing and having an **emotional psychological well-being** allows a person to develop a stronger capacity for personal growth, showing signs of a positive attitude in spite of the circumstances or situations we are going through.

When a person develops this level of consciousness, they feel good and calmer, knowing that they are in control of their emotions and are able to cope with the pressures of everyday life, which is the basis for a healthy, happy, and fulfilling life.

Emotional psychological well-being is the key to overcoming all psychological-mental limitations. The poor understanding of what we human beings really are, limits the person to experience a life full of joy, but when you open yourself to this understanding, at the same time you are opening yourself to personal growth and development, allowing you to establish new effective and satisfactory relationships with others, with yourself and, especially, with your own thoughts.

Happiness or feeling happy is a temporary state of mind, it is just one more of all the emotions and feelings that human beings experience during their lives, such as: sadness, loneliness, anger, discouragement, courage, peace, love, tranquility, etc.

All these emotions and feelings are necessary for human beings. Without them we would not be able to live to the fullest this wonderful experience we call life. Although eternal happiness only exists in movies, television shows, and children's stories.

By this I do not mean that we are destined to live unhappy lives.

Achieving a better lifestyle is possible as long as we are willing to change the paradigms we have taken for granted until today.

It is necessary for humanity to discover and open itself to a new way of living life to the fullest with its ups and downs, joys, and sorrows; to change that way of thinking that human beings came to this world to suffer in order to earn something, but on the contrary, every human being has the right to live a life full of love, peace, and prosperity.

Everything that happens to us in life is just part of the human experience that we live as individuals. Since childhood we are taught countless paradigms, methods, ideas, theories, and lies about happiness. For example: it is necessary to have millions in bank accounts, properties all over the world, and the newest cars, or to have all the material things you want in order to be happy.

One of the most important paradigms that we must change in order to achieve a fulfilling life experience full of satisfaction and without limitations here on earth is that we need to be aware of what our true essence is, what our mission is and what we were brought into the world for, in other words, to give a true purpose to our existence.

Discover how human beings relate to each other and how you are the creator of your own story. Understanding this will fill you with a new understanding and guide you to seek new ways of living.

The self-improvement coaching of the human experience and together with the studies and discoveries of neuroscience made by doctors, psychologists, and scientists, will lead you to have a clear understanding of the above mentioned.

Precisely, the objective of this book is to help us understand the life experience with a different perspective, changing the paradigms that limit us to reach our goals.

I have tried to write it in a simple, practical, and short way because it is not necessary to be a psychologist or to have a master's degree to be able to understand how your brain, mind, thoughts, and emotions work.

I deeply believe that all people can achieve great things because within each one of them dwells a being much bigger and more powerful than their human limitations, since all human beings relate to each other through our thoughts and that is where the limitation of the human being often lies.

Remember, depending on how you relate to your

thoughts, so will be your experience of life with others and with the world around you.

Brain and mind

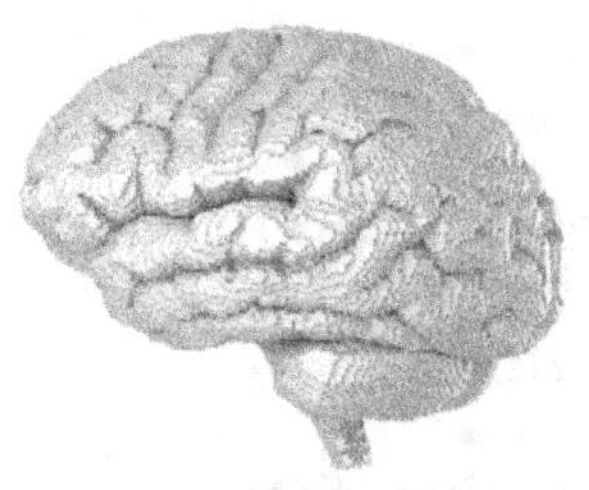

I AM NOT
THE ONE YOU THINK I AM,
Because I
I AM THE ONE WHO THINKS

Index

1.- WHY DIDN'T ANYONE TELL ME THIS BEFORE?

Maybe when you read this book you can relate to it, maybe at this moment you find yourself in depression, with no will to live, with fear or with very high levels of anxiety.

You have to recognize that life holds no grudge against you, because we are the ones who take for granted that problems or situations are bigger than our greatness.

There is no problem or situation bigger than you, depending on what you believe as true, you give life to those situations from your thoughts, because that's how your brain perceives it. That is why there is nothing wrong with us, all those thoughts of guilt, fear, depression, anxiety, or stress lead you to experience emotions and feelings, but they are only creations of our brain, the one who decides to believe them as truth is you.

The dissatisfaction you feel with life is creating a situation of searching for something else and that is very important to notice. Keep in mind that you are not alone, thousands of people are in the same situation as you and that is what led me to look for a new way of living life.

When I was most confused and frustrated, unable to find a single solution to my problems, tired of dragging a limitless amount of guilt from my past, frustrated for not being able to achieve happiness and after having exhausted all my strength I only thought that there was no more to do, when suddenly, from inside me, a thought of struggle arose and I said to myself "there has to be something else, I cannot give up", then I began to search the Internet for methods of self-improvement and that's where the magic began.

The personal transformation coaching of the three principles turned my life around, led me to discover who I really am, my true identity and how I function as a human being; I understood that it depends on the relationship I have with my thoughts. I am creating my own life experience.

Why wasn't I taught that there is a different way to live life?

I believe it is not time to judge the past, it is time to change the present and look for what has been hidden.

That is why I did not stop there and decided to continue the search. I met with great psychologists, doctors, and teachers who teach and study the subject of the functioning of human beings, I mean, neuroscience.

All this knowledge brought a new beginning to my life and the more I learned, the more clarity I gained. I began to look around me and realized how people go through life like zombies without knowing what they are looking for. It was here that I decided to write this book and put its context in an easy-to-understand way and share it to the world so that more and more people discover their inner potential, reach their goals, and have a better lifestyle.

I want you to keep in mind that what I propose here is not about religion or sects, it is an invitation to enter, discover, analyze and understand the various behaviors of human beings, starting from their thoughts, emotions, and, of course, without leaving their spirituality aside.

Giving a true and new meaning to life will lead you to look at the world from a different perspective, freeing you from many misconceptions.

I have no doubt that you can achieve what you want in

life, you just need to propose it to your mind, because, just as it helped me, I know it will be of great help to anyone who is willing to change the rules of the game, in other words, to be willing to stop being the piece of the game and become the player of their own story.

This proposal that I share with you is a practical and simple way to live and understand life, developing a better human experience without limitations, without taking anything personal; remember, life holds no grudge against you, it only depends on how you relate to different situations and so will be that experience.

Life has its ups and downs. We cannot deny this, but there will always be a light at the end of the tunnel, the night does not last twenty-four hours, and after a storm the sky always clears. No matter what you are going through right now, everything is temporary, whether it is a personal, emotional, financial problem, or illness.

We have great examples of people who, despite the circumstances in which they lived, managed to emerge victorious from those situations, and you will not be the exception.

For example, Viktor Emil Frankl, a neurologist,

psychiatrist, philosopher, writer, and Holocaust survivor, never gave up despite the difficult situation he had to live through.

Viktor E. Frankl's phrases make a lot of sense for those who are looking for a new way of living.

"Our greatest human freedom is that,
despite our physical situation
in life,
we are always free to choose
our thoughts.

When we cannot change a situation,
we are challenged to change ourselves."

-Viktor E. Frankl.

Since our childhood we have been programmed to live a lifestyle full of lies, carrying a list of erroneous ideas that limit us to have a full life experience. We have been taught to look for happiness on the outside when true well-being comes from within us, from our inner spiritual self.

Humanity needs to open itself to the search for inner well-being, which will lead to the understanding of the true purpose of life.

In the brain of the human being, where the magic of the human experience has its origin, is where our mind dwells, whose job is to give life to thoughts. It is there where your human experience begins and it all depends on how you relate to your thoughts will give place to a group of feelings and emotions that will trigger a reaction in your body, it is precisely there where each individual creates their personal life experience.

There is no other way to create life experience because human beings relate to each other through thoughts, depending on the relationship you have with them, you and only you will be the creator of your own life experience. In other words, you are the only creator of your story, no one can change the way you see life but you. Outside situations have no effect on you if you do not allow them to.

The greatest mistake of human beings is to believe that there is something wrong within us that must be corrected, when the only thing that must be corrected is how we relate to our own thoughts.

Now the big question is: **Why didn't anyone tell me before?**

I believe it's never too late to start, so get ready to change big paradigms that you don't even know you have taken for granted.

One of the greatest mistakes of human beings is not recognizing that we have made mistakes and that sometimes we make the wrong decisions, but at the time we thought it was the only way.

Let's not judge our past decisions because it makes no sense to go back there, life does not judge you for what you did or did not do, you are the one who puts yourself in judgment, life is not complicated, but we make it complicated, now is the time to act, to straighten what is crooked and start a life full of wellbeing.

I invite you to enter together into a new world where you will find your missing connection

"The greatest mistake of human beings
was to desire to separate the human from the
spiritual,
which was impossible.

There can be no human experience
if we do not have a body and a spirit;
however, a link
can put it all back together again.

Spirit and matter are necessary
to achieve a human life experience.

Once the spirit leaves matter
returns to its pure essence:
Spirit. "

-Víctor Arreola.

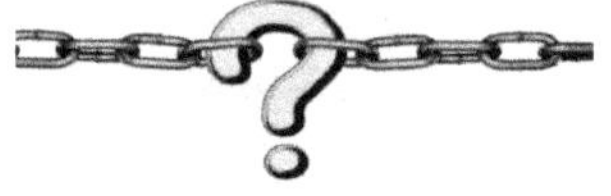

2.- BE WILLING TO RELEARN

What do I mean when I mention being willing to relearn? The Dictionary of the Spanish Language says that the word "reaprender" (relearn) comes from the Latin reprehenderé and means "to correct, to call attention to disapprove a fact".

Precisely, that is what we need to do, to correct what we have been taught for many years and that many times we are not even aware that we are validating that idea that was imposed on us since our childhood.

Now is the time to relearn to live life with a different perspective and new ideas. It is necessary to free ourselves from all those things that limit us from being able to have a better lifestyle and achieve a high psychological well-being.

Little by little you will discover all those ideas that you have taken for granted, but they are just that, "ideas", and you have validated them as absolute truth.

For example: having a distinguished social standard of living so that society respects you or having a professional career to achieve happiness. Thinking that we are bad and need to suffer to deserve something good in this world. All of the above are just a list of ideas that do not allow a person to reach their full potential.

It is necessary to change these paradigms that take us nowhere because the only thing they do is to put limitations on our shoulders, making us believe that life must be a journey full of pain and suffering.

Changing some paradigms can be a bit difficult for many, because having to face their own ideas, culture, religion, or dogmas can create an inner conflict in any person, since for a long time each one of them has been believed as an absolute truth.

Then you might be asking yourself: **"How to start relearning?"**

First of all, you have to recognize that each one of them are just that, ideas or beliefs that our ancestors, as our parents or grandparents taught us and imposed them as the only truth, it is good to be aware that someone also imposed those same beliefs on them, and they did not realize it. So we do not have to reproach them because that is what they were taught.

And, therefore, that was taught to you, and you have

validated it as true for all this time and it has been your absolute truth until today.

Don't try to change everything from one moment to the next or to confront those beliefs or ideas. It may take you some time to reflect and discover what is true for you. Take as much time as you need.

Each human being is unique and therefore my reality may not be yours. The only thing you have to do is to be willing to open to a new understanding and that you gradually identify each one of them.

Put them on trial and find out if they help you grow as a human being or if they are limiting you from having a better life experience.

This is a great step that you have taken until today. Just giving yourself the opportunity to analyze each one of them is a great challenge that you will achieve little by little. Many of us did not even realize that we had so many ideas, beliefs, and taboos in our lives.

Remember, the fish does not realize it lives in the water until it is taken out of there.

Thus, we did not know that there was a different way

of living until someone had the courage to open the door to the wisdom of the human being.

The human brain has the capacity to adapt to new situations or lifestyles, thanks to its neuroplasticity.

WHO (1982) defines the term "neuroplasticity" as the ability of cells of the nervous system to regenerate anatomically and functionally after being subjected to pathological, environmental, or developmental influences, including trauma and disease.

I ask you to take some time for reflection and with the following questions identify what are those ideas, beliefs, taboos, or stories that you have validated and that you have believed as absolute truth in your life until today.

Take the time to answer these questions from your inner self and analyze each one of them:

1. What was it that you were taught as a child that you sometimes question whether it is true or not?

2. How willing are you to change the paradigms in your life?

3. Do you remember which experiences have marked your life, for better or worse?

4. Is there someone or something that hurt you in your childhood?

5. Have the memories of that experience marked your life?

6. Do you think the past will define your future?

7. Are you satisfied with your goals and life experience?

8. What are your fears in life?

9. What goals would you like to achieve?

10. What limits you in achieving your goals?

I ask that after each chapter you go back and ask yourself these same questions, I want you to realize how each one will change the way you think.

3.- BEING TRULY PRESENT

Being truly present is vital in order to get the most out of this piece of work, this is not a book to simply read, but to deepen into all its contents.

Has it ever happened to you that sometimes you are in the car driving and, at the same time, you are thinking about other things you have to do? You are everywhere but driving the car, as if it was on autopilot and already knew where you wanted to go, you have arrived at your destination, and you did not even notice what was going on around you.

The same thing happens to all of us, we are thinking about things of the past or the future, we are mentally running all over the place as if our compass did not work and we forget a very important detail: the present, the now, we overlook it, and tomorrow we will suffer because we will be longing for it.

Unfortunately, this way of living has become a vicious cycle and many of us don't even realize it.

During the industrial era it was promoted that people should multitask, that is: have the ability to do two or more things at the same time. We were led to believe that developing this ability was to have a good mental development, which is totally false.

One more example: when you decide to prepare a cup of coffee while you heat the water and put the coffee in the cup, several thoughts go through your mind, you are mentally in another place, less present in preparing your cup of coffee, that's how we are all used to doing everything, automatically.

Right now you can be reading this book and at the same time be thinking about something you didn't do or have to do later.

Mankind is focused on living in the past, in what they did not do or should have done, remembering something that has already happened and is not relevant in the present. This will often lead the person to depression.

Another type of person may live worried about the future, filling themselves with anxiety. Our brain processes about sixty thousand thoughts a day; more than ninety percent of them are repetitive and about eighty percent of them are negative thoughts.

That is why I emphasize the importance of being truly present and not letting ourselves be carried away by the number of thoughts that our brain experiences.

> "YESTERDAY IS HISTORY,
> THE FUTURE IS A MYSTERY,
> BUT TODAY IS A GIFT,
> THAT'S WHY IT'S CALLED THE PRESENT!"
>
> -OOGWAY.

We overlook the present (gift) because we are everywhere but in the here and now. I invite you to practice being truly present. Today, when you talk to someone, stop whatever you are doing and give them your full attention, stay with that person one hundred percent, I mean, stop wandering with your thoughts.

Human beings spend their time remembering the past and wishing for the future, which leads them to experience feelings of depression and stress while they are not even aware of the present.

Remembering the past or thinking about the future is not a bad thing, but we run the risk that these thoughts and emotions become chronic without realizing it and we end up depending on pharmaceuticals and antidepressants.

Of course this is big business for the big pharmaceutical corporations, they would like you to get to this point of being dependent on them because that is a million-dollar-business for them.

The COVID-19 pandemic alone caused a twenty-five percent increase in anxiety and depression worldwide.

I am going to ask you for a moment to STOP TO THE RUNNING OF YOUR DAY TO DAY and give yourself a few minutes for you, the world will not stop because you are not running after it, humanity will follow its course, do not doubt it. Put a brake on the running of thoughts and observe your present.

I invite you to put all those things that worry you aside for a moment. Take some time to live your present; take a deep breath and notice all the people around you, clear your mind of all worries, this will give you more clarity to make better decisions in life.

"When we live in automatic
we move away from our present
and when we no longer have it,
we yearn to go back there.

Don't cry for the past,
nor yearn for the future;
live in the present while you can,
seek no more what you have not lost,
enjoy the greatest gift you have ever been given:
life.
Enjoy it now that you have it,
even with its ups and downs."
-Víctor Arreola.

4.- FINDING YOURSELF

Finding yourself is very important for psychological wellbeing and many times this is where all the confusion of the human being originates; I ask you to reflect on the following questions:

1. **How can a person claim to love another person if they do not love themselves?**

2. **How can you take care of someone if you don't take care of yourself?**

3. **How can a blind man guide a blind man?**

In this last question I am not referring to a person who is visually impaired, but to the person who goes through life aimlessly and purposelessly without knowing what they were brought into the world for or where they are going. Our teachers in life (our parents) taught us what they were taught as well.

I remember once I asked a great woman if she knew what her mission here on earth was, she was a fighter, intelligent, full of love, extraordinary; she had seven children and in times of economic crisis she managed to feed them all, always taking care of them even with all those limitations, and she knew how to take care of them, supporting her husband in everything. Sadly, she answered me: "I don't think I had any mission here on Earth". That answer was very sad for me.

How sad and empty life can be for people who spend their time without recognizing what their mission is.

I want everyone who reads this book to be able to find themselves, their inner natural essence, and I invite you to do it now.

Take a mirror in your hands and stare into it,

what do you see?
Who do you see there?

Don't look at the human being you have always thought you are, look at the being that lives inside you, the one who has no name, the one who has no limits to love and be happy, the one who is willing to forgive, the one who can give everything for others no matter the cost. That being, the spiritual one you look at there, that is the one you truly are.

Do you know why that being can give everything?

Because that being you see there is an expression of the Creator who can do everything, even to the point of giving life to a being made of mud and water like you and me. That Creator Being, who is like an immense ocean, and we are a drop of Himself.

That is why your greatness is as great as the greatness of the being who created you. Call Him God, Abba, Yahweh, Adonai, Jehovah, Eloah, Creator, Omnipotent, King of kings, or simply call Him as you want.

We are made of matter, and we were given a spirit which gives us life. I do not intend to enter into religions or beliefs, this I leave to your discretion and inner intelligence. My intention is to invite you to change this paradigm, to discover it from within.

Find yourself.

> "The natural essence
> of the human being is Love,
> but when you get carried away
> by thoughts of hatred and rancor,
> is corrupted
> and self-destructs itself. "
>
> -Víctor Arreola.

5.- THE TRUE ESSENCE OF THE HUMAN BEING

For decades we have had a wrong idea of who we really are, where we come from and where we are going. Humanity tried to separate the matter from the spiritual in us, which led us to the biggest mistake. There can be no human life experience if there is no spirit and body together.

In some cultures it is believed that having bad or negative thoughts makes us bad people, others believe that having bad or negative thoughts offends our creator.

According to recent scientific studies, it is estimated that we have about sixty thousand thoughts a day, ninety percent are repetitive, and eighty percent are negative. If this were true, we would all be bad or negative beings.

This is not a bad thing, this is simply the way we human beings function, our brain is the most complex organ to study because that is where our thoughts and emotions originate, but it depends on how your relationship with your thoughts is, so will be your life experience.

How can you make a lemon stop giving lemons if that is what it was created for, but with lemon juice you can make a sweet lemonade.

We humans were created to be able to experience life to the fullest, and just because we have so many negative thoughts does not mean that we have to be negative about everything, because we have free will, in other words, we are free to decide what we want to do and how we want to behave. Remember that eighty percent are negative, but you have twenty percent positive thoughts.

If we analyze it in depth, we can only come to the conclusion that it depends on how your thoughts are or with what kind of thoughts you relate to, so will be your emotions which will lead you to have certain behaviors, and from there will determine your performance in life, both personal, familiar, and professional.

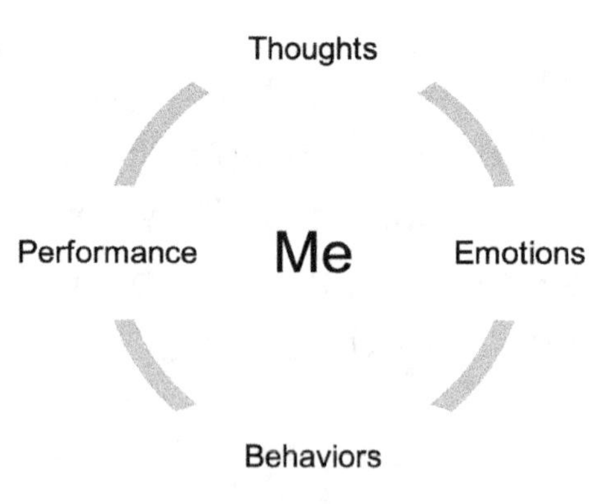

Another idea that we were taught is that achieving material goods and creating fortune on earth will lead us to happiness, that is why we are running every second to achieve our goals without taking into account our present, and if for some reason things do not go as we think, we fall into disillusionment or depression.

This is because, for centuries, mankind has had a wrong idea of who we humans really are. We were called earthly beings as if we were truly eternal on this planet called earth, and we spend our lives in pursuit of material goods thinking that when we have them we will be happy.

Has it ever happened to you that sometimes you wish you had something like a house, a car, a professional career, or something material, and you think that when you have it, you will finally be happy?

But what happens after you achieve it after a short time? There is still that emptiness inside you, that emotion of happiness disappears and that is not bad because experiencing happiness is only a temporary state, but psychological well-being is a way of life because even if you are going through a problem or a difficult situation, you know that everything will pass and that you will be fine at the end.

Of course I believe that there is a superior being, the creator of all things visible and invisible, and it is He who allows us to have this human experience here on earth.

A being who is an immense ocean of love, peace, truth, and life and you, a small drop of that ocean of love, you are His expression of love here on earth.

That is why it must be clear who you really are. You, a living expression on earth of that being, you, the greatest proof of His love; that is your essence.

Here I would like to emphasize that no matter what happened to you in your childhood or what could hurt you during your life, but there is something in you that no one can touch and that is your essence, because that essence belongs only to Him, to that being who gave you life, and I am not referring to your father or mother, but to your Creator, the one who holds you when you can no longer, the one who cries and smiles with you, **God, Abba, Yahweh, Adonai, Jehovah, Eloah, Creator, Omnipotent.**

All these are just words that can't begin to describe

how infinite, great, and wonderful our Creator is.

He does not make bad people, but human beings get carried away by those negative thoughts that our human brain sends us, but always keep in mind that you have the ability to ignore them and let yourself be carried away by the immense love that dwells within you.

Humanity lacks nothing to reach its full potential, it only needs to get rid of its bad thoughts, let them pass without taking them into account.

It is like the story of the caterpillar that becomes a butterfly, it is not that it becomes a butterfly, but only that it gets rid of what hinders it to be able to fly.

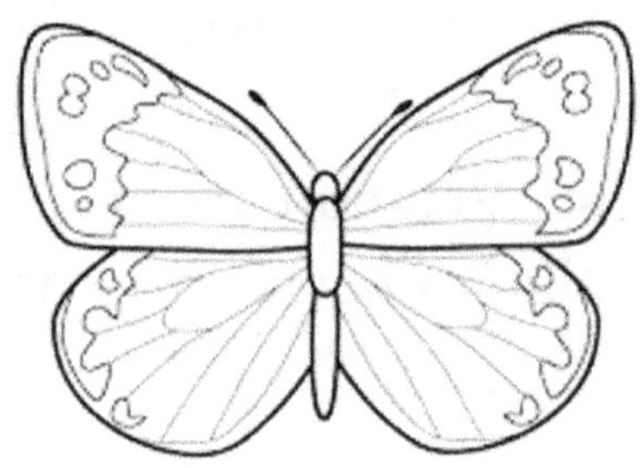

"Fear is the greatest enemy.
of the human being,
but if you don't stop being a caterpillar,
you will never be able to spread your wings
and fly.

If you are not willing to discover
who you really are,
you will be left crawling on the floor
as the caterpillar.

Dare
and you will fly very high, so high
that you will soon reach the top. "

-Víctor Arreola.

6.- CHANGING PARADIGMS

As we already talked a little in chapter 2 about the need to change some paradigms, I would like to make it very clear that in order to achieve psychological wellbeing it is necessary to change what we have always taken for granted and has created a limitation for us to realize ourselves as human beings.

Many of these paradigms only create a mental noise that disturbs us. In the world there is only one absolute truth, and that is that we are all spiritual beings having a life experience here on earth, and in a not-too-distant time this experience will come to an end. The life experience is gone in the blink of an eye.

Open yourself to change all those limiting paradigms and replace them with others that will help you build a future full of achievements and satisfactions, since they are just ideas that someone proposed and that got validated by a group of people.

I invite you to make a list of paradigms, ideas, or beliefs that you would like to change. Identify them and reflect on why you want to change them and how they are affecting your life.

7.- WHERE DO OUR THOUGHTS, FEELINGS, AND EMOTIONS ORIGINATE?

The brain is the organ or apparatus inside our head, and it is the cradle of all our thoughts, remember that our brain sends an average of sixty thousand thoughts a day, of which, ninety percent are repetitive, eighty percent are negative and only twenty percent are positive, but our brain does not know how to distinguish if they are bad or good, it only creates them.

The mind is in charge of giving life to those thoughts, that is the stage where the magic begins. When the mind gives life to that character that the brain proposed as a thought, that provokes a reaction in us.

Every thought in action brings with it a feeling, and the feeling can create an emotion which, as I mentioned before, will trigger a reaction in our body, more specifically in our nervous system, which makes us feel strong or vulnerable, depending on the relationship I am having with that thought, there is nothing wrong with this, it is part of our survival system.

Another paradigm that we must change is that every

feeling or emotion is generated in the heart. This is false, thoughts, feelings and emotions are created in our brain through hormonal changes in the nervous and endocrine system, which is responsible for regulating hormonal changes in the human body.

The nervous system is made up of the brain, brain stem, cerebellum, spinal cord, peripheral and vegetative nervous system.

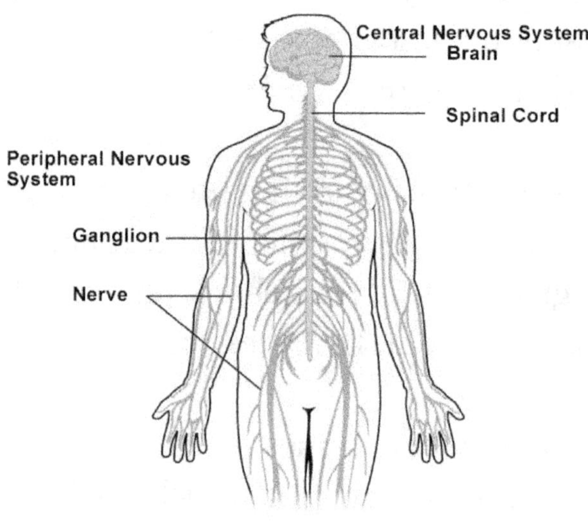

The endocrine system consists of the hypothalamus, pituitary, thyroid, parathyroid, adrenal, pancreas, ovaries and testes.

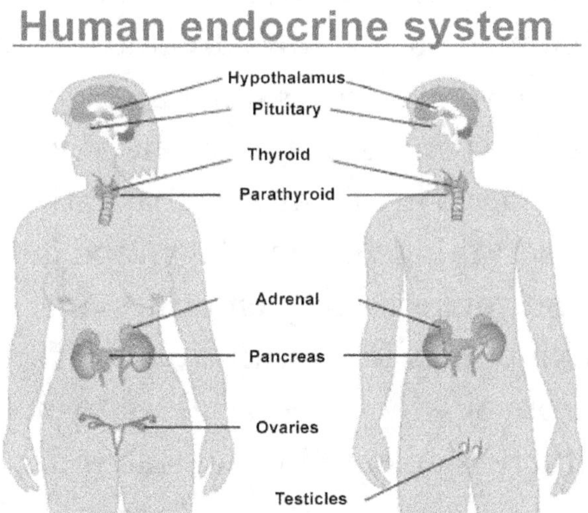

8.-PERCEPTION OR REALITY

Think for a moment that you've managed to get that school diploma you've always dreamed of, that you've gotten the job you've always wanted, that you've found your prince charming or the queen of your dreams. You have achieved in life what you have always wanted, you have everything, but one day in the morning you wake up and you feel a deep emptiness inside you that you don't know how to fill with. You don't know where it comes from or why you feel this way, you have it all; however, there is an emptiness inside you.

Have you ever believed the story that when you get what you want, you will be happy? Then, where does happiness originate? Why this emptiness?

Sometimes we, human beings, think that happiness comes from the things, situations or people around us, when in reality all the emotions we experience are created within ourselves.

Our brain is only capable of capturing 5% of all the information that surrounds us, and of that 5% our brain is only aware of ten percent, which means that we create our reality from only 0.5% of all the information that surrounds us. This 0.5% is what each person uses to know if they like or dislike something or someone. When your brain sends a thought it is only using that small percentage to produce that proposition and is leaving out 99.5% of your true reality.

People's daily lives are made up of thoughts, emotions, feelings and perceptions, and that is where we create our reality, but it is all a person's perception.

It is how I perceive it with that 0.5% and from there I make it my reality, but this does not mean that it is the same reality to others.

Think for a moment about a situation you are going through right now and look with this understanding at it. **Are you using only 0.5% of the information? Do you feel it in your nervous system as a reality? Are you aware that what you are feeling is due to how you are perceiving it from your mind?**

Remember that your brain is only sending the proposal, your mind is perceiving it and you are the one who is giving it that interpretation. Just because you interpret it that way does not mean that it is an absolute truth because you are leaving out 99.5% of the information.

This happens to all of us, it is not only to you, that is why I say that there is nothing wrong with being human, it is simply to recognize what kind of relationship we are having with our own thoughts, because remember that at any moment we create our reality and it depends on how is the relationship with your thoughts, so will be your life experience.

I ask you to reflect on this before moving on to the next chapter.

9.-WHY SHOULD WE CARE ABOUT WHAT WE THINK AND TAKE FOR GRANTED?

As I have already mentioned before, each of the thoughts we believe as truth or we validate bring with them a reaction in our body, and that is why we must be very careful in what we think and take for granted.

If we look around us we can find people who live worried and stressed all the time, there is nothing wrong with worrying about a situation, but it becomes a problem when this way of relating to our thoughts becomes chronic.

The causes of chronic stress can be numerous, but basically it can be said to be those unresolved situations or many times they are just negative thoughts that are maintained for weeks, months or even years.

It is very easy for these people to worry because they are always looking for a reason to feel attacked and to be able to excuse their stress. The worst thing is that, if left unchecked, stress can reach a pathological level of anxiety that causes major disorders in the body such as: increased heart rate, high blood pressure, diabetes, obesity, menstrual problems, sleep disturbances, constipation, diarrhea, headaches, sexual dysfunction, irritability, mood swings, fatigue, feeling weak, difficulty breathing, memory problems, fatigue, panic attacks, weakening of the immune system, and easy-to-get infections.

The human being was created to live in harmony, peace and tranquility, but only we alter the hormones in our body. This, together with all its organs, is regulated by the brain. The nervous system is in charge of conducting signals between neurons and coordinating all the actions of the body.

When the person experiences a moment of tension, whether real or imagined, the **sympathetic nervous system** is activated and, therefore, the heart rate increases, there is a change in the contractions of the heart muscle and it widens (dilates) the airways to facilitate breathing, causes the organism to release stored energy and muscle strength increases. This is also known as the survival nervous system.

On the other hand, we have the person who tries to see life with a different perspective, a little more positive, using twenty percent of positive thoughts, the nervous system that is activated is the **parasympathetic**

nervous system that slows the heart, dilates the blood vessels, reduces the size of the pupil, increases the digestive juices and relaxes the muscles of the digestive system.

This nervous system also begins to function when the person has already passed a state of anxiety, so it creates in the organs and in the body a state of calm when the danger has culminated.

Taking care of what we think and what we take for truth plays a very important role in our health and our lifestyle, because when we are stressed cortisol levels rise affecting our health.

Doctors of neurology say that continued high levels of cortisol can cause a person's health to begin to deteriorate on several levels causing health problems by suppressing the immune system, altering metabolism and causing the person to be more likely to have diabetes, osteoporosis, chronic fatigue and weight gain.

Remember that what harms the human being is not what goes in, but what comes out of them.

"Practicing forgiveness
compassion and
charity,
helps to maintain
thoughts under control
and, therefore, we can experience
a better life experience and well-being.

Hatred and rancor
do not harm the other person,
but to the one who carries it inside. "

-Víctor Arreola.

10.- HOW TO START HAVING A BETTER PSYCHOLOGICAL WELL-BEING

Practically, you have already begun to generate this change in you, by allowing yourself to enter into this new understanding you have already begun and it does not matter if you return to that automatic pilot because this happens to all of us, but when a situation presents itself to you I am certain that your inner intelligence will remind you of what you have learned so far. Remember, there are two ways to live life:

The first is to be the chip in the game. What do I mean by this? Well, it is that when the person lives in this way he becomes so vulnerable, that everything that happens around him has a direct effect on his life because he gets carried away by the situations of the outside world creating a pessimistic world inside him directly from his thoughts. When you feel that you are here you must leave as quickly as possible, remember that you are creating this situation yourself through the negative thoughts that your brain is proposing and you are validating them.

The second is to be the player. In this form, the person decides who to give permission to enter his life and create a relationship of thoughts, has it ever happened to you that another person tries to make you angry, but you are in a level of tranquility so high that it does not get you out of there, simply because you do not feel like getting angry with anyone? That level of psychological well-being is what you should reach and if for some reason you give permission to the other person to make you angry, you always have the option to get out of there and return to your natural state of tranquility, remember that everything is in the way you perceive the situation and you relate to it from your thoughts.

Also start by changing those habits that create conflicts within you, avoid meetings with negative people, eat healthy, do some exercise such as walking, practice meditation such as *mindfulness*. All this will help your nervous system to rehabilitate and get used to this new way of living and achieve freedom in your thoughts.

"Achieving a life experience without
limitations is your decision.

The limitations you have to overcome are
your own thoughts.

Thoughts are just proposals of your brain
and do not mean that they are true.

People are not in control of your life
if you do not allow them to do so.

You build your life experience moment by
moment.

Live life instead of thinking about it.

You are the creator of your own story. "

-Víctor Arreola.

11.-WHAT IS MINDFULNESS?

Mindfulness is a meditation technique that consists of observing reality in the present moment of the here and now, without judgment and with full openness and acceptance.

Its objective is to achieve a deep state of consciousness free of judgments about our sensations, feelings or thoughts, to pay attention to what is happening inside us at every moment.

Here are some easy exercises to perform in your daily life.

Exercise 1: One Minute of Mindfulness

This is an easy exercise that you can do at any time of the day and in any position you want. The goal is to focus all your attention on your breathing for one minute.

Keep your eyes open, breathe in through your nose and let the air enter your belly instead of your chest and expel the air that comes out through your mouth. Focus on the sound and rhythm of the breath. Be prepared for other thoughts to cross your mind, watch them go away and slowly bring your attention back to your breathing, and do the same each time this happens. At the end of the minute stretch your body as much as you can and yawn through your mouth.

You can do this exercise as many times as you want, as it helps you to restore your mind, get clarity and peace.

This exercise is the fundamental basis of a correct mindfulness meditation technique.

Exercise 2: Conscious observation

Choose an object. Any everyday object: a coffee cup, a pen, a crucifix, a candle, etc. Now allow your full attention to be drawn to this object. Just observe it. Keep your breathing at a normal rhythm, let your body do the breathing.

Bring your full attention and feel the sensation that you are fully awake and aware that you are here at this moment. Notice how the mind frees itself from thoughts and focuses on the present moment. It is subtle but powerful.

You can also practice conscious observation with

your ears by playing music and closing your eyes. Sometimes listening is much more powerful than watching.

Exercise 3: Count to 10

This exercise is very similar to exercise 1.

Only, in this case, instead of focusing on breathing, you have to close your eyes and focus your attention on counting slowly to ten.

If at any time you lose concentration, you must return to counting by number 1. In most cases it goes something like this:

Example: "One... two... three... I have to buy milk today. Oh, no, I'm thinking" You stop and restart counting "One... two... three... four... I thought it was easier to stop thinking... That's a thought! You have to start over... One... two... three... now I've got it. I'm really concentrating now...". Try to do that for at least one five minutes.

Exercise 4: Observe your thoughts

It is difficult to get any stressed and busy person who

leads a fast-paced life to give it up to focus on a stream of thought through the mind.

The idea of sitting down even causes them more stress. If you are one of those people, instead of working against the voice in your head, you can sit and "observe" your thoughts instead of engaging in them.

In this way you will not be able to eliminate them as in the rest of the exercises, but it is a good technique to reduce their intensity.

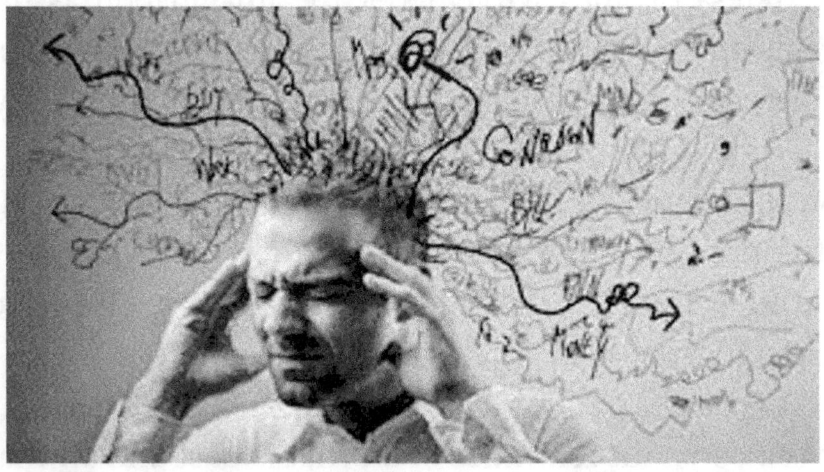

TO STOP THINKING IS IMPOSSIBLE. It is the nature of the mind to perform this action, that is why we are rational beings. Welcome to the human experience.

12.- TURN DOWN THE VOLUME ON YOUR MENTAL NOISE

It is necessary to lower the intensity of your own judgments that you make towards others and towards yourself. That inner voice disguised as fear, of what people will say, of making you feel inferior and incapable of achieving what you have always wanted, are just thoughts and proposals from your brain. **Mental noise is just a bunch of thoughts inside our mind**.

St. Teresa of Jesus wrote about the imagination as the madwoman of the house, referring to the chattering or inner dialogue of thought that drains our energy uselessly.

Buddha spoke of a monkey constantly demanding our attention, jumping from branch to branch, pointing out to us the fears in it, alerting us, shrieking for us to listen to them.

It is a constant reminder of all that is past and all that is future that comes to destabilize us, remind us of our failures and anticipate our catastrophes.

Jump and jump, branch to branch, negative thought to negative thought.

> "YESTERDAY IS HISTORY,
>
> THE FUTURE IS A MYSTERY,
>
> BUT TODAY IS A GIFT,
>
> THAT'S WHY IT'S CALLED THE PRESENT."
>
> -OOGWAY.

LIVE YOUR LIFE TO THE FULLEST AND WITHOUT LIMITATIONS